15 Mistakes People Make When Seeking Knee Pain Treatment

_____

How to Avoid Surgery

Dr. Olesnicky and Dr. Hashimoto

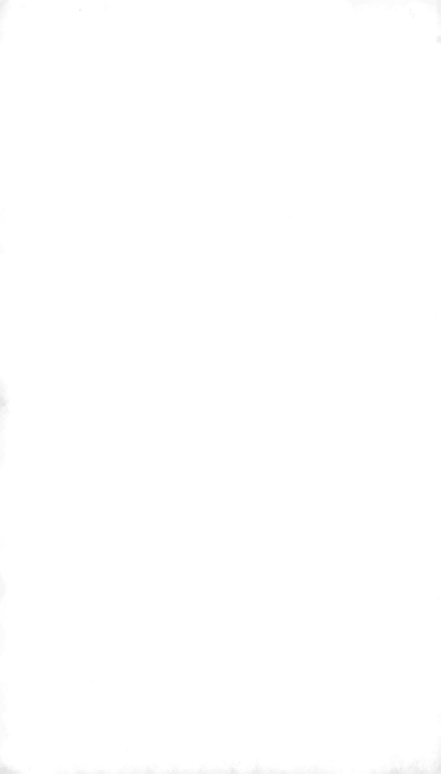

First Edition

ISBN 978-1508441434

Printed in the United States of America

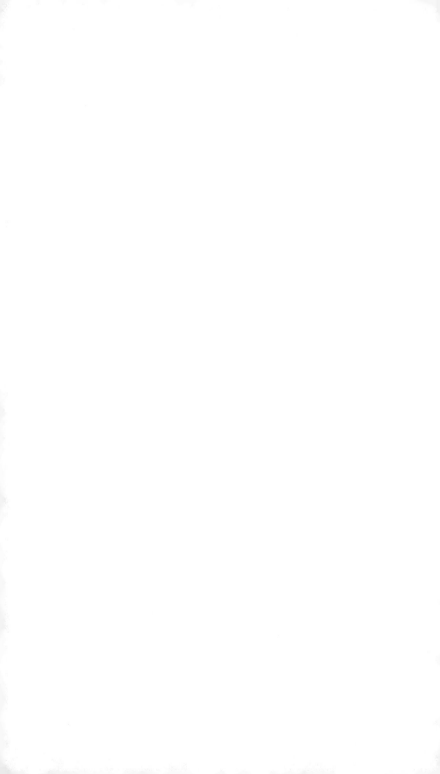

Table of Contents

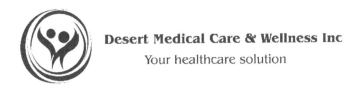

Desert Medical Care & Wellness Inc
Your healthcare solution

Introduction

At Desert Medical Care & Wellness we understand, you hate this. You hate everything there is about pain and dealing with the pain. You hate going to doctors, waiting and getting outrageous bills for what felt like a little bit of service.

There are the cases where you or a friend who have gone to one or more doctors and have come out worse than you were before going in.

Our goal at Desert Medical Care & Wellness is to give you the best information we can about your pain and what treatment options there are available, along with the associated costs, benefits and risks.

Ultimately, life without pain and a body that moves properly so you can do the things you desire is an investment in YOURSELF.

Being in pain will physically and emotionally drain you and affect your overall outlook on life and what you choose to participate in.

With the exception of the next page, this guide is not about us, it is about you. And should you decide to receive treatment from us we will be honored that you trust us enough to improve your health and wellbeing.

But if not, we hope that helping you avoid these 15 major mistakes regarding pain relief will get you back to your life as soon as possible.

To your health and happiness from Drs. Olesnicky & Hashimoto.

Who Are Dr. Olesnicky & Dr. Hashimoto?

Dr. Hashimoto and Dr. Olesnicky's mission is to help as many people as possible to reach their full health potential in the Coachella

Valley. Both of them started their healthcare journeys because they ultimately wanted to help people. However, it doesn't take long before any doctor starts seeing the gaps in care

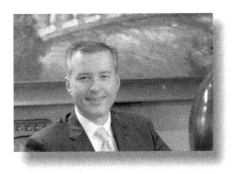

we have in our society and that there is no quick fix.

Dr. Olesnicky is the son of two physicians and started out as an emergency medical technician prior to going to medical school. He spent his childhood in Eastern Europe, but moved to the US when he was a teenager which is why he speaks not only fluent English and Ukrainian and also some Russian, Polish and German. Working in the emergency room is where he enjoys practicing but he also holds a board certification in internal medicine as well.

He has always seen value and results combining traditional and progressive medical

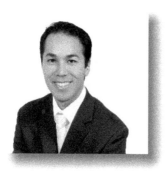

care with acupuncture, chiropractic and physical therapy which is why he teamed up with Dr. Hashimoto.

Dr. Hashimoto started his career in pre-dental but after a severe car accident that did not resolve during 6 months of physical therapy and pain medication he tried chiropractic before his visit with an orthopedic surgeon. He was amazed with his results. He quickly changed career paths and enrolled in Southern California University of Health Sciences for a Chiropractic Specialty his next semester.

Practicing in the desert Dr. Hashimoto understood that even with all the therapies his office used he was still limited with regards to treating some of the advanced degenerative arthritic conditions he faced. Working with Dr. Olesnicky was a natural fit.

Their core passion is health and wellness which includes pain relief but there is much more to health than just being pain free.

Their goal for you and the goal of this book is to enable you to really understand all the factors of knee pain and why working on the entire body provides long lasting results that is healthy.

After all if you could eliminate some dangerous medications, steroid shots or surgery why wouldn't you?

This book will finally help you solve your knee pain problems.

Chapter 1: Knee Pain 101

Do you dread walking down stairs?

Getting up from your seat after a long car ride or going to the theatre?

Are you always looking for an elevator?

Does it hurt so bad that it affects the quality of your life?

Are you starting to feel old?

You are not alone! Knee pain is one of the most prevalent complaints in America. And it's no joke. Knee pain can take a lot of the joy out of life, make work impossible and render one helpless.

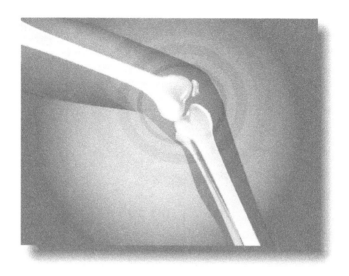

What is exactly is Knee Pain and what are the best natural methods to give you relief from your pain?

Knee pain can strike at any time, *15 Mistakes People Make When Seeking Knee Pain Treatment* details a unique method of reversing knee symptoms by removing numerous triggers as well as toxins by using a natural process.

This is a simple, powerful & natural self-treatment process which borrows its formulation directly from tried and tested facts as well as age old remedies.

Bring your knees the highest level possible of muscular strength, flexibility, and endurance!

In this book you will find what the best natural remedies are to treat your condition. You'll discover the following:

• A better understanding of knee pain.

• How to keep knee pain from getting worse.

• A simple weight loss method that will help you lose 12-25 pounds per month.

• Remove certain foods from your life and see results in days.

• Find out the best alternative medicines and treatments that can help you.

• What will improve your strength and help with the pain.

• How to cope with knee pain so that you can still perform important daily tasks.

• Know what type of exercise can give you relief

from the symptoms of knee pain.

• What type of supplements you can take to treat your condition.

• Step by step knee pain treatment for relief.

Knee pain can range from minor discomfort that acts as a mere nuisance, to excruciating debilitation. The symptoms vary based on specific issues being experienced in each case, but mobility generally decreases as the severity of knee symptoms worsen.

Various types of arthritis, mechanical problems, and other interacting factors can all play a role in determining the extent and duration of the knee symptoms experienced by each person. There are various levels of knee pain, as well as many different types.

Although there are over 100 varying types of arthritis, with the knee, osteoarthritis is the most common. This form of arthritis results from gradual deterioration as age and use start to wear away at the cartilage of the knees.

Other types of arthritis such as the autoimmune condition known as rheumatoid arthritis may pose more debilitating concerns than osteoarthritis, but more people are affected by osteoarthritis of the knees than other types of knee arthritis.

Additionally, mechanical problems can affect knee pain as well. Iliotibial (IT) band syndrome is a common mechanical issue which frequently plagues endurance runners.

The IT Band which originates on the outside of the pelvic bone and inserts on the outer portion of the tibia becomes excessively tight and begins to rub against the femur.

Hip or foot pain can indicate mechanical issues related to knee problems as well, since discomfort in these connecting body parts can cause the sufferer to compensate accordingly with altered movements in gait and other motions which may impose greater stress on the knee joint.

Perhaps the most important mechanical issue related to knee pain is a misaligned kneecap in which the triangular patella which covers the front of the knee is jarred out of place.

This patellar slippage usually occurs to the lateral or outside region of the knee joint, and can often be readily observed as a dislocation as the kneecap remains displaced from its proper position in front of the knee.

Correcting knee tracking issues can make a big difference in reducing pain and improving range of motion.

Incorrect tracking is a sign that the knee joint is not properly aligned and re-aligning the knee will lead to proper tracking which is something we will discuss later in this book.

With regards to knee pain, there are a number of risk factors which contribute to the likelihood of such pain occurring.

Obesity is a major issue in this case.

Since the knees must support the bulk of a person's body mass, any additional weight will cause the knees to take on a greater workload, stressing them excessively in the process.

The more weight on the knees, the less they will be able to remain in good working order for a long duration. Combating obesity by exercising and eating healthy in order to lose weight and maintain this lower body mass can be very beneficial for people experiencing knee pain.

Previous injuries are a cause for concern as well. Once one injury has taken place, the propensity for future injuries is heightened accordingly.

The same issue may recur in some cases, while other issues may sometimes pop up as well due to compensation for previous injuries that cause a person to alter the way he or she moves.

Finally, repetitive use can also be a contributing risk factor.

The human body is designed for movement, but it is not designed to continually perform the same repetitive tasks over and over again without proper rest and time for recovery.

Many people are subjected to repetitive conditions at work or elsewhere, and this repetitive stress can wear down the knees over time, leading to chronic knee pain associated with a variety of issues.

These and other interacting factors also serve as complicating factors due to the convoluted relationships between the interactions of these risk factors.

Chapter 2: Alignment

Mistake #1: Alignment Matters

Do your ankles cave in or fall out when you stand and walk?

Are you bowlegged?

Do your knees cave inward (aka knock knees)?

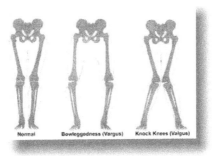

Regarding the knee that is hurting, does your ankle, hip or back hurt on that same leg? What about the opposite leg?

If you answer yes to any of these, make a HUGE note of that!

Look at the diagram below to see how everything is connected. Your pain may be stemming from your ankle and settling in the knee.

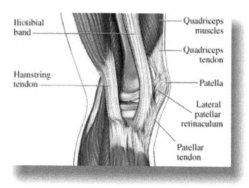

Or it could be from a quadricep muscle knot that's embedded deep inside the muscle.

An unaligned muscle with tension build up could be the pain (common). It could be from the Iliotibial Band or IT Band (most common).

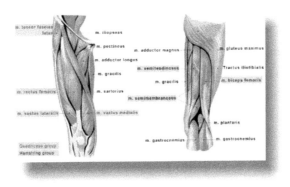

By finding the movement during which you feel the most pain, we can follow its route through the body, pin-point source and eliminate your pain with proper corrective measures.

Q Angle

The Q angle of the knee is a measurement of the angle between the quadriceps muscles and the patella tendon and provides useful information about the alignment of the knee joint.

These are basic examples of natural alignment issues that are all very common in women. It is also very common for these to cause knee pain as well as hip and back pain in many people.

There is no denying the connection between

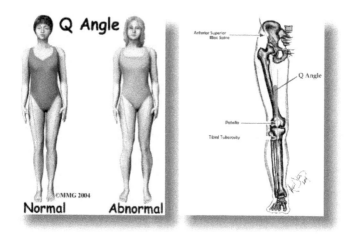

knee, hip and back
pain. They are all related, which is why a knee problem will travel up to your back if you do not address it.

Does this sound like you? Pain in your hip that aggravates low back pain? Poor balance? Feeling like you run out of space between you and the ball on your golf swing (leading to slicing and/or hooking)?

What about your attitude towards things you used to enjoy?

Can you still do simple things like walk up stairs or get in and out of a car without having to prepare yourself?

There's a lot to know about this, so bear with me. There is hope for you yet.

Chapter 3: Why Check Above And Below The Knee? Your Butt and Ankle Matter

Mistake #2: Skipping The Glutes

How do your butt muscles contribute to your knee pain?

These are the stabilizers of the body. Your body's balance is controlled by these muscles. In my professional opinion, the glutes are the most important muscles in the body. Yet, they are

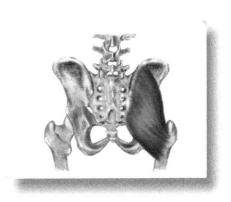

also the laziest muscle in the body.

These muscles tends to be inhibited and I feel that this probably began when humans started sitting in chairs.

We sit on our glutes all day long and eventually they begin to become inhibited or "lazy". This problem doesn't exist in cultures that squat rather than sitting in chairs, which is why proper sitting ergonomics and exercise can make a big difference for knee pain.

The glutes have two main parts: The gluteus maximus and gluteus medius. Both are important and play a role in solving the knee pain riddle.

The first thing I always do is make sure the muscles can fire.

Surprisingly, they do not pass this test in about 99% of the patients who have knee or back pain.

Strength vs. Activation

It doesn't matter if you appear to have big muscles, activation is important because if your muscle doesn't fire when it is supposed to fire, there is no point in having a strong muscle.

This is a mistake that most make with exercise. They value strength over activation. But activation trumps strength every day of the week.

Strength is related to how much power, weight or force your muscles can generate to move an object or perform a task.

Activation is your body's ability to fire when necessary like when you step, jump, get out of a chair or just get up from the ground. When these muscles do not fire at the appropriate time, your body is smart enough to recruit adjacent muscles in order to perform the movement your body is attempting to make.

This is a how a lot of problems develop because when another muscle takes over like that, two things will happen:

First, when adjacent muscles fire that are not true stabilizers, it will likely change the biomechanics in that area. This will lead to increased wear and tear because the joint is NOT moving through its normal motion.

Second, when the muscles compensate, those muscles have taken up a second job and begin to get over worked. This leads to muscle spasms/cramps initially and eventually as the muscle fatigues you will begin to develop more adhesions and trigger points in those muscles.

This is why many patients will say they benefit from deep tissue massage, but I'll talk about fascia, adhesions and trigger points in a later chapter.

Your glutes need to fire when they are supposed to!

The main reason is for proper biomechanics of your legs and knees.

These muscles will prevent your thighs from rotating inwards which leads to 'knock knees' and torqueing of inside part of your knee.

This in turn leads to increased wear and tear on the medial (inside) part of your knees.

Not coincidentally, the medial part of the knee happens to be where 90% of knee osteo-arthritis is located.

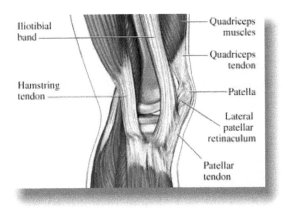

When your thighs rotate inwards it also stretches out your Iliotibial Band (ITB) on the lateral side of your thigh.

This will increase the amount of friction in your hip bursae.

Many patients that suffer from lateral hip pain and bursitis will have a problem with this issue.

If you are a golfer, this will lead to slicing and/or hooking the ball.

But That's Not All...

The problem doesn't stop there either, now that your knees have rotated internally,

- This will internally rotate your shin bone (tibia)...
- Which creates a misalignment in your ankle...
- Which causes your ankles to roll inwards and your arches to flatten (also called flat feet or over pronation)...
- Resulting in your ankle losing balance ability, which is bad for walking and sports...
- It will also lose flexibility.
- With a stiff and immobile ankle this will create excess mobility in your metatarsals, and...

- This leads to the dropping of your metatarsals...
- Which can contribute to pain in the balls of your feet as well...
- A stiff ankle will put also more stress on the knee. When you squat, walk or bend your ankle and hip have to bend along with the knee. If you have reduced motion in the ankle, hip and spine, this will put more stress on the knee.
- Also resulting in flat feet...
- Which may lead to plantar fasciitis (foot pain/inflammation) ...
- And now that the feet are flat this will change the biomechanics of the feet and big toe...
- Which means the big toe will not flex as well because the toe has rotated inwards...
- This can lead to bunions and big toe pain.

Wow! That's quite a lot of cause and effect.

These are reasons why so many patients benefit from properly fitted foot orthotics, which will correct the flattened arch and will partially untorque your leg and pelvis.

One of the reasons why our advanced non-surgical knee treatment system works so well, is because we treat adjacent movement systems such as the foot/ankle and hip/pelvis.

We even get results with patients who have been told they were bone on bone and had no other options other than surgery

Just like a door with three hinges, if you remove two hinges from the door, the third one picks up the additional stress and will warp. When most people get knee pain, they will only receive treatment for the knee because that is how insurance and our healthcare system works.

You must treat the area of complaint when working with insurance.

This means rehab and injections for the knee. But no treatment for the hips or ankles.

Most will get a shot of cortisone for knee pain because this will remove the inflammation and your pain but it will not fix the problem and the steroid will actually accelerate the decay in that joint.

More about this later.

I apologize about the tangent that I have taken you, but I had to make sure you understood.

I hope I made the case as to why glute activation is essential for any knee, back, hip and even ankle rehabilitation program.

If this is not part of your physical therapy program, I hope it is because you don't need it and not because of your insurance or an omission by your doctor.

Foot Placement

Step in some mud then go for a walk. Look at the foot imprint you leave behind. Do all the points of contact of the foot show up? Or are their some spots of your foot missing? More than likely, you have some spotted foot imprints showing up on the pavement.

This is totally normal, but also totally imbalanced, and a reason behind knee pain.

Earlier, I told you why over-pronation decreases ankle mobility and will increase stress on the knee, and this is easy to see with a

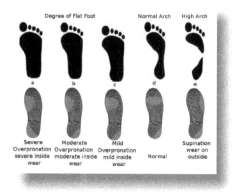

foot imprint, shoe wear pattern or assessing how you walk (gait pattern).

If your complete arch touches the ground like the picture above on the left, then your foot is too flat.

If your wear pattern on the ball of your shoe is on the inside portion only, then you probably over pronate, if the crease on the top of the shoe where your toes flex is on an angle you probably over-pronate.

Normal wear on your shoe is with some on the lateral-posterior portion of your shoe and even wear on the ball of your feet, with a straight shoe crease on top of the shoe in the toe box area.

If you are unsure if you have this problem, just bring in a pair of shoes to our office.

Make sure they have been worn for 6 months. With that we will give you a free gait consultation to see if you could benefit from this unique type of treatment.

Chapter 4: Correcting "Knock Knees" (A Large Q-Angle)

I told you why glute and muscle activation is important and now it's time to learn how to activate muscles.

Part 1: Activate

The glutes are inactive in most patients, which is why I start by teaching patients how to activate their lateral and posterior glutes (gluteus medius and maximus).

This helps with alignment, stabilization, balance and rotation of the femur (thigh bone). A weak glute will cause internal rotation and torque on the knee and flattening of the arch in the foot because it is needed for stabilization.

This is why I always look at the pelvis for any knee or back problems.

Activation is hard to teach in a book, but a simple method you can try at home is to lay flat on your back and put your hands under each butt cheek. Now try to fire off each butt muscle individually without firing anything else, especially your hamstrings.

Once you can do this easily, try doing the same in other positions.

This is a basic exercise that is taught prior to any advanced movement because activating the muscles in the appropriate order does matter with knee pain.

Part 2: Strengthen

These are your typical exercises such as bridges, squats, getting out of a chair, etc. I have listed some of these exercises in the exercise section with some photos in a later chapter.

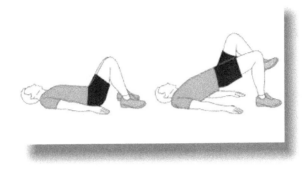

Typical advanced exercises include firing off the full glute at the same time. This can be done with a single leg bridge or body weight squats with resistance bands around the thighs. The band fires off the lateral glute and squat fires off the posterior glute.

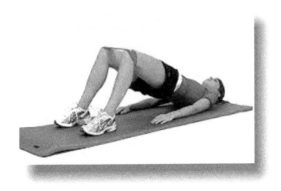

Part 3: Mobilize The Tissue And Joints

The foam roller and therapy stick are key pieces of equipment for "self-massage" or breaking up adhesions in the muscles.

These tight knots develop in the muscle when it is over worked and under stretched for a long period of time.

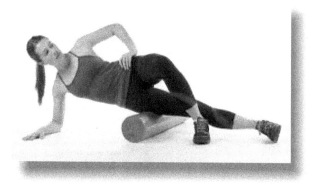

I always suggest rolling over the glutes, lateral thigh (ITB), front (quadriceps) and back (hamstrings) with the foam roller.

Then I suggest rolling over the inner thigh (adductors) and calves down to the ankle with the therapy stick.

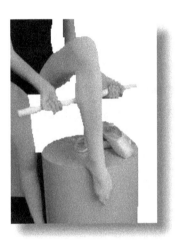

If patients have difficulty using the foam roller, I just have the patients roll up and down the leg with the therapy stick.

This is basically like a light rolling pin, with many wheels on the stick used to roll out the knots in your muscles.

This is followed up with stretching of the tight muscles and mobilization of stiff joints.

The reason why we care about stiff joints and tight muscles is because this reduces flexibility.

 If you have knee pain, it is important that surrounding tissue and joints have mobility.

The reason for this is that if the surrounding tissue and joints around the knee must be mobile otherwise you will put too much stress on a knee that is already failing.

Chapter 5: Common Mistakes in Physical Therapy, Medication and With Injections.

Mistake #3: Chasing Pain – The Problem with Physical Therapy

To be clear, I'm not saying that where you feel pain or that the actions that create pain don't matter.

They actually matter a lot, but too many doctors and therapists spend their careers chasing pain.

That means if you have pain in your knee, the entire examination, all of the diagnostic tests and the treatment are done on the knee.

This seems to make sense – but it is too narrow a view.

My three hinge analogy explains this extremely well, because medicine and many physical therapy prescriptions are focused on the remaining hinge instead of also optimizing the adjacent hinges.

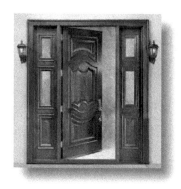

Part of the time this is because the medical doctor didn't think to examine the other areas, but one of the most major reasons is that insurance *only pays for areas of complaint.*

In this case the knee.

So chasing pain is built into the system. Not broader diagnosis. A diagnostic test done on the hip when it is the knee that is hurting will be considered an unnecessary test and will be denied. The doctor will also possibly be looked at as someone who is trying to defraud the insurance company.

Now that you understand that everything is connected and that knee pain could really originate from a pelvic or ankle problem, you will be able to understand why the prescription for physical therapy could be written incorrectly.

Most knee pain patients will start out on their knee pain treatments with their primary care physician. In fact, this is one of the top 10 reasons why anyone will see their family doctor.

A primary care doctor must know about many different conditions, pains and many other things including medications which is why it is impossible for them to be experts on muscle, bones and joint pain (orthopedics).

In real world terms, this means if you have knee pain, you will get medication and physical therapy written for that knee pain.

The physical therapist is expected to focus on the knee and not the ankle, pelvis, spine, etc. Sometimes this is the reason a patient does not improve despite physical therapy.

Even if physical therapy is done on the correct area, most treatment is focused on rehabilitation of the muscles and very little is spent on proper joint re-alignment.

Consider a whole body approach before surgery if this method of "knee only" treatment doesn't work for you.

Mistake #4: Avoiding Joint Manipulation Because You Are Scared Of Getting Cracked

Not too long ago if you had a clogged coronary artery or rotator cuff tear it would require a surgeon to either break open your chest or make a large incision in your shoulder.

Technology has evolved and now arthroscopic surgery exists. Those large scars are replaced by three tiny scars where scopes and devices are inserted into the body to perform the surgery.

Manual chiropractic manipulation has existed since 1895 and it is still used today. It works well in many cases but technology makes things easier.

There are impulse devices that will send small but precise shockwaves into the joint or tissue at a high frequency that will loosen up a joint without having to 'crack' or 'pop' the bones.

If you have brittle bones, arthritic joints or fear of having your joints popped this is a very good option for you.

Hands on and instrument mobilization will provide the safest and longest lasting maximal range of motion of your joints in your legs and pelvis.

When re-enforced with exercises mentioned in the exercise chapter this will produce excellent outcomes.

Mistake #5: Placing All Of Your Eggs In The Diagnostic Test Basket.

Knee evaluations tend to be based on consultation and diagnostic testing only. MRIs will commonly show arthritis and meniscus wear that will be a main focal point by the medical provider.

The diagnosis often ends with that one test rather than performing a careful physical and orthopedic examination of the knee and adjacent areas, combined with what YOU, the patient, tells them.

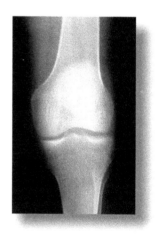

Too many times providers place the entire weight of the diagnosis and the treatment on the diagnostic tests.

Doctors forget about the functional and physical exam of the joint combined with what you, as the patient, have to say about what hurts, what doesn't, what your balance is like etc.

I'm not saying x-rays and MRIs are not important, I just like seeing other examinations performed along with them where knee pain is involved.

When you consider the complex nature of the cause and effect factors that can bring about knee pain – it only stands to reason that a doctor should look beyond that one area.

Mistake #6: Pain Management with No Attempt at Structural Correction - Why Drugs and Cortisone Can Be a Problem In The Long Run

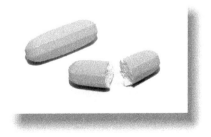

There are far too many people who seek treatment for their knee pain symptoms rather than looking for the true cause of their knee pain. Many patients end up treating themselves with over the counter medications.

This practice can be very dangerous.

Nonsteroidal anti-inflammatories (sold as Advil, Aleve and a under great many other names) alone contribute to over 100,000 hospitalizations per year at an estimated cost of $15,000-$20,000 per case. This leads to 10,000-20,000 deaths per year and is the 15th leading cause of death in the USA, so this should be taken seriously.

These stats are rising and probably have gone up since this data was reported in in the early 2000's. Just to put this in perspective, fewer than 14,000 people died from AIDS in 2011 and I'm sure you have seen plenty of media attention and public service announcements towards this disease.

NSAIDS are an effective method for treating arthritis pain, but taking these on a regular basis can wreak havoc on your kidneys and digestive tract.

Many people will get regular or periodic cortisone shots which are steroid injections in the knee joint. While this is often very effective at reducing inflammation and pain for acute knee pain, it is not a good idea for long term knee pain.

Providing immediate therapy and mobilization of the knee and adjacent structures while this inflammation and pain is reduced is useful but if you are getting these shots done and skipping out on the exercises, this is probably not your best long term solution.

To help you understand why I feel this way about long term use of cortisone shots let me explain to you how it works. I'm going to get slightly technical, but bear with me as I try and break it down for you.

Cortisone Shots

Cortisone is categorized as a glucocorticoid or corticosteroid. So yes, this drug is a steroid, but it's not exactly the kind that has been circulating in major league baseball. Glucocorticoids, including cortisol, are produced naturally in our bodies to manage glucose metabolism, growth, and stress by breaking down muscle into glucose. Glucose = sugar = energy source.

These natural steroids also help to limit inflammation. Under stressful situations, our bodies release more cortisol, which increases circulating glucose and limits the ability for muscle and fat cells to take glucose in, thus blood sugars rise. Glucose is a ready energy source and prepares us for increased activity to handle stress.

Glucocorticoids are also immunosuppressive, which also helps to explain why it is anti-inflammatory, because inflammation is an immune response. The man-made variety of glucocorticoids, which includes cortisone, are powerful anti-inflammatory drugs that are delivered in a larger quantity than the body produces normally in order to provide therapeutic benefits for certain diseases.

My patients usually ask me about using cortisone for the management of different types of arthritis or inflamed soft tissues, such as bursitis.

So, how does it relieve pain? Inflammation causes pain. Cortisone works by altering the genetic material in certain cells which causes them to stop releasing the chemicals that cause inflammation and limit damage to the surrounding structures.

It also decreases swelling by constricting the surrounding blood vessels thus limiting their ability to take on more fluid.

No more inflammation = no more cranky, swollen joints.

Side Effects

There are many side effects to taking glucocorticoids. Here are the biggies:

- It breaks down things in our body that contain collagen, which include: muscles, bones, ligaments, and the skin.

This can lead to myopathies, which cause muscle wasting and weakness. Also, increased risk of osteoporosis

- Increased risk of developing infection because it suppresses the immune system.

- Increased risk of developing peptic ulcer.

- Increased risk of developing glaucoma.

- Diabetics take note of this side effect: Hyperglycemia, insulin resistance, decreased control of blood glucose.

- Mood changes.

- Hypertension or High blood pressure.

- Your body's natural processes for making glucocorticoids may be suppressed.

So, how do I feel about cortisone injections?

Since the medication is administered locally at the joint where you want to limit inflammation, it is less likely to affect other areas of the body, unlike an oral medication.

Cortisone is highly effective at decreasing pain in most people in the short term. If pain is controlled, your therapist can start to work on areas of the body that can help to reduce joint stress and limit the progression of your disease.

Also, because cortisone breaks down muscle and bone, it is even more important to come to therapy and work on your strength.

If you get cortisone shots a couple times a year or have for many years, I wouldn't worry about the above risk factors since long term use of oral medications are the only methods that could cause all seven.

However, the breakdown of tissue, collagen, ligaments and bone is a realistic problem in your joint if you keep getting cortisone shots in your joints for many years.

What About Surgery?

Before opting for surgery and subjecting yourself to the complications and potential issues that can arise during and after going under the knife, you should consider your other options.

Surgeries can be successful in some cases, but there are many instances in which surgery is neither the safest nor the most effective option.

First of all, there isn't really such a thing as a minor surgery. All surgical operations carry an inherent degree of risk. This risk varies, and you of course would not expect a relatively non-invasive surgery of the knee to bring the same degree of risk as open heart surgery, but the risks are always present.

Even when an operation is carried out by a knowledgeable and experienced surgeon (which, hopefully, should always be the case) there is still the potential for future complications following the procedure itself.

Traumatic injuries and even repetitive stress can exacerbate injuries that have been repaired by surgery, potentially necessitating further treatment even after recovering from the initial surgery in the first place.

Knee replacements are liable to failure, and there are other options which should first be considered before choosing surgery.

Therapeutic remedies like basic physiotherapy can often resolve lingering issues that might otherwise require more drastic treatment such as surgical operations to repair damage.

Ideally, reaching the proper compromise of strength and flexibility of the knee joint can fix knee issues before these issues end up requiring surgery.

Importantly, the knee should not be looked at strictly in isolation from the rest of the body.

Knee issues can impact, and be impacted by, other factors relating to body mechanics and structure.

Gait issues, hamstring, gluteal, hip flexor, and even back problems can all contribute to knee discomfort, and potentially impede the recovery process.

By ensuring things are strong enough and not too tight, you can promote the proper alignment in your joints that allows your knees to function smoothly over the long term.

Fixing issues before they become major problems can be a main key to avoiding surgery, and if such options are available then they should generally be considered before committing to surgery.

Hip and foot pain can often be a warning sign of knee issues so if something seems wrong with other parts of your body then you may still need to consider the knee issues potentially contributing to the pain you are experiencing.

Everything is connected and if you can focus on ensuring the proper function of each body part then you can better ensure that your knees will promote health and longevity throughout the rest of your body.

Issues related to a lack of mobility and range of motion are often best addressed with the methods mentioned in this book.

Although surgery may be helpful and even required in extreme cases, there are often safer alternatives which prevent the knee pain sufferer from subjecting themselves to the risks of going under the knife for a potentially unnecessary surgery.

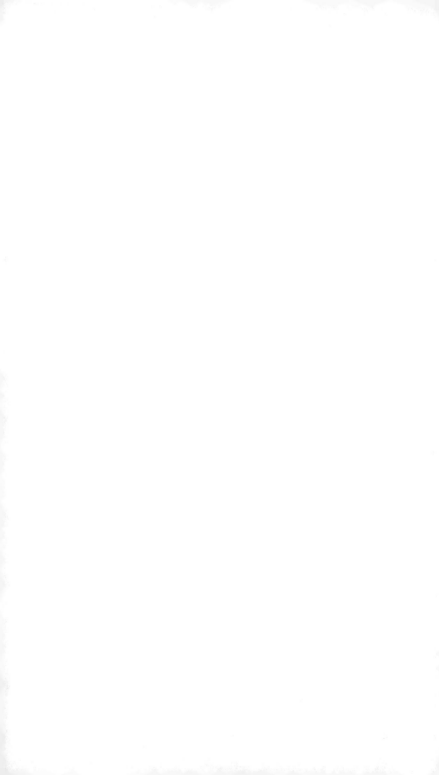

Chapter 6: Why Does Health Care Cost So Much in This Country?

Knee pain or any type of pain is just a symptom, and this is your body's warning signal that something is wrong.

What do I mean by that? Symptoms tell you something is wrong in your body. Have you ever had an upset stomach? Your body was telling you something.

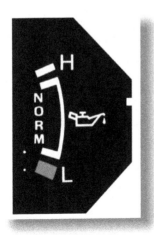

Here's another way to look at it:

If you're driving down the highway and your oil light comes on, or your oil gauge reads ZERO, that probably means something is wrong with your engine.

It means you should stop driving the car.

IMMEDIATELY!

Otherwise you're going to have an engine that will burn itself up for lack of oil.

This RED oil light turning on or oil gauge showing oil pressure has dropped is just a "symptom".

It's not the problem.

Your engine's oil level or the pump that creates oil pressure is the problem.

The oil light/gauge is the symptom.

It's just letting you know something is WRONG. That's all. You don't need a new gauge.

Your body is no different. When you start to have achiness and pain those are symptoms.

Drugs cover up symptoms.

For example: If your RED oil light goes on or the oil gauge shows ZERO, do you pull over and cut the wire?

No you don't. Why would you do that? The RED light or the oil gauge is your car's system trying to tell you that your engine is having oil issues and is in imminent danger of damage.

Your Body Is Doing The Same Thing!

Your symptoms are not the problem. Stop trying to get rid of the symptoms with medications. You can use medications to help your symptoms while you're taking care of your problem, but don't think getting rid of your symptoms is FIXING your problem. It's not!!

Think about this. If NO signals were sent, you could be in pain from infection or burning yourself, but you wouldn't realize it because your nerves were no longer sending signals,

So symptoms are good.

The reason why this is costly is because the problem never gets addressed, and if this progresses too long it will eventually progress into a larger problem that only surgery can address - which is extremely costly.

If the surgery does not correct the problem, you may need another surgery or a lifetime of therapy or pain management to manage the problem.

As you see, medical costs begin to add up quickly, which is the number one reason why our medical system costs so much to run, because we focus on symptom control and emergency care rather than prevention.

Mistake #7: Avoiding Synergistic Therapies Because Of Potential Costs or Time?

Avoiding synergistic therapies because you thought it would cost more or it would be inconvenient.

If you wanted to get into shape you wouldn't just stick with running or yoga or weight lifting or just diet, you would integrate multiple things together to get the best results.

So why would you just stick with a one size fits all approach to healthcare?

Many people go to physical therapy and get great exercises and stretches but don't get therapy like hyaluronic acid joint injection. Or they miss out on acupuncture, laser or joint work like they do at the chiropractor.

It is not uncommon to have muscle, joint and nerve problems that can be best addressed by multiple techniques, which is why some providers will refer you out to different offices for different types of treatments.

However, wouldn't it be nice to go to one office and get one type of treatment and when you are done just pick up your bag and move into the next room to see the other doctor?

I have personally treated thousands of patients and have seen many difficult cases that have failed in acupuncture, chiropractic, medical treatments (injections/medications), pain management and physical therapy prior to coming to our office.

There is nothing special about the water in our office and we don't have a magic wand despite what some of our raving fans say. One of our secrets is integrating just the right amount of different types of therapies.

By providing a unique blend of therapies rather than trying to fit you into a ONE SIZE FITS ALL approach we can achieve BETTER RESULTS in a timely fashion.

Mistake #8: Only Focusing On Structure

How many times have I had patients come into our office suffering from knee pain who were told to lose weight, but were not told how to lose weight?

Too many to count.

Simply incorporating some minor nutritional changes can lead to a dramatic improvement.

For example if you are overweight and suffer from knee pain, simply by addressing your weight problem you will decrease your incidence of knee pain.

If you are overweight, a simple weight reduction of 10% of your total weight will more than likely reduce some or all of your knee pain - if it is a minor case.

Dr. Messner performed a study that showed that one could reduce up to four pounds of force off each knee by reducing body weight by one pound.

Our office will incorporate a weight loss program with anyone who is overweight that will reduce weight by 12-25 pounds in 30 days and 24-50 pounds in 60 days. This is typically more than enough for all of our knee pain patients.

To learn more about this please pick up a copy of Dr. Hashimoto's book, *7 Mistakes That Women (and men) Over 40 Make When Trying To Lose Weight*. This book discusses, among other things, why hormone imbalances can contribute to weight gain along with how one can reduce weight quickly by harnessing the power of your hormones.

Even if you don't need to lose a lot of weight, just the reduction of specific foods such as grains, sugars, dairy, starches and bad fats reduces inflammation.

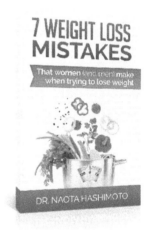

If you feel better after taking Ibuprofen, Motrin, Aleve or other Non-Steroidal-Anti-Inflammatories (NSAIDS) then you will improve by converting to a whole-food, non-inflammatory diet.

Doing so will probably decrease your level of pain and accelerate the rate that you will heal. Inflammation will exacerbate any condition and can create some diseases. As a general rule, anytime you reduce inflammation, your body will respond in a positive manner.

Even if you don't quite buy all of that - I am pretty sure you will agree that part of the healing process means that you have to have the right building blocks to repair your injury. Big Macs might taste good but they will not supply your body with the appropriate ingredients to facilitate the healing process.

If you know that your overall health is not what it should be and your doctor doesn't guide you in the right direction then you may be in the wrong office or may need a referral for co-treatment from a provider that does.

What supplements should I take?

Our office uses a proprietary blend of pre-digested, whole food supplements for inflammation, joint repair and pain relief.

Our inflammation support actually out performed 600mg of ibuprofen in a double blind study.

These products are optimal for people over the age of 50 because they are pre-digested, all natural and loaded with natural enzymes which make them extremely bioavailable in your body (meaning that you actually absorb the nutrients).

Many patients have asked me about joint supplements and some patients will swear by a brand while others will say it didn't work for them.

This is because some people do not digest their nutrients well and joint supplements and herbs are especially difficult to digest. This is why I highly recommend our joint support formula to anyone over the age of 50. Even if your digestive system is perfect, why not consume a product that is absorbed at 100% rather than something as low as 30%.

Mistake #9: Only Sticking With What Your Insurance Covers

If you wish to be on the cutting edge, sticking with insurance is not what is best for the patient. This is because insurance typically covers drugs or natural therapies and new devices take time before they are added to an insurance plan.

It's not because these devices don't work, or don't have research behind them, they just may be too new. However, if you have an HMO or another poor quality insurance company you will get substandard care in the medical office.

HMOs, ACAs (Affordable Care Act Insurance) and other substandard insurance plans are able to offer a plan to you as a discount because they severely reduce reimbursements to providers and limit what tests and treatments they can provide.

Guess who will have a shortened treatment time when they need help?

Of course, it will be the person with the bad insurance. In fact, with HMO insurance most doctors get paid a flat fee to accept that HMO plan and they will actually lose money by providing too much care for too many HMO patients. Typically the goal is to provide good enough care to keep the HMO happy, but not too much that the doctor's business is not profitable anymore.

I'm not going to lie to you about healthcare, it is a business, just like any other business and if the business is no longer profitable the office will eventually go out of business. Most medical clinics and providers start with great intentions of helping patients like you, but unfortunately there is more and more pressure put on doctors. That starts with student loans.

The cost of medical, chiropractic or physical therapy school increases every year and so does the cost of living. Reimbursement to providers has steadily declined over the years and the amount of fighting an office has to do with an insurance company is only increasing.

Most insurance companies will automatically deny 20% of perfectly submitted insurance claims because they know providers like us don't have time to follow up on all the bills sent out. This leads to an increased cost in running a medical office because we need more staff to chase down bills and fight with insurance companies. That leads to pressure to see more patients by the doctor and decreased quality of care.

So why am I spending time discussing this with you? The point I am trying to make is that sometimes your insurance company is not your best friend and sometimes you need to try things that may not be covered 100% by your insurance to get the quality of care you deserve.

Our office uses as much insurance as possible, but since we offer some services that are not covered by insurance companies, we don't have to spend as much time chasing down insurance checks. Which means less overhead and a calm doctor who is focused on you rather than the 8 people in the waiting room who were supposed to have been seen 15 minutes ago.

Chapter 7: Star Trek Medical to the Coachella Valley

What Could Laser (Light) Therapy Do For Me?

Light therapy is not a new concept. The sun's photonic rays have the power to cause a seed to sprout through tiny biological changes. These rays are called full-spectrum, which means that it is made up a wide range of non-specific wavelengths.

Out of all those many wave lengths, there is only one that causes that seed to sprout (germinate).

If you don't care about the technical information, please skip the next 7 paragraphs.

Ninety years ago, Einstein predicted the common use of lasers, which stands for Light Amplification by Stimulated Emission of Radiation.

Since that time there have been many scientists working on this new idea of laser technology and how it can affect a biological organism. In 1978 there was the Wave Particle Theory, which has been used to discover which frequencies and wavelengths would communicate with different parts of your body, i.e. your skin, muscle, ligament, etc.

Traditionally lasers had been used in surgery to cut tissue but recently their use has been redirected toward regenerative uses (that is, eliminating pain and promoting healing).

Laser therapy is based on photochemical and photobiological effects of the cells and tissues. With laser light, cell function is stimulated, especially the ability of a cell to create a special chemical called ATP (used by the cells to create the energy that runs them).

This increase in ATP is associated with increased cell metabolism, the increased manufacture of collagen, stimulation of DNA formation, stimulation of the immune system and an increased new formation of capillary blood vessels.

Certain lasers also have been shown to increase neurotransmitters (serotonin), to increase and enhance tissue regeneration through increasing both fibroblasts and keratinocytes (cells important to repairing injured tissues), and to also increase antioxidants.

All of this works to accelerate bone and scar healing.

What that means in plain English is that the laser delivers deep, penetrating, photonic (that is, light) energy which creates changes that help to repair damaged areas of your body and promotes healing.

The result is a decrease in pain, a decrease of inflammation (swelling) and true healing. These laser treatments are cumulative, so it is not uncommon to cut the healing time in half for injuries and completely eliminate pain associated with these injuries.

This laser approach is also a great therapy for old chronic injuries, because certain lasers have the ability to break up old adhesions and scar tissues from past injuries and surgeries. If these were injuries were causing pain, then the pain will likely go away.

Deep tissue laser therapy does not require the use of neither drugs nor surgery, and there are no known negative side effects or risks associated with these laser treatments, as there frequently are with other forms of treatment.

There are a wide variety of lasers out there, some are non-specific in what they can be used for, while they may provide some benefit only the high quality medical grade lasers consistently show the highest and best results.

There are a number of different grades of medical lasers, all of which are approved for this use by the FDA: A Class III laser or "Cold Laser" is a low level.

On the other hand, Class IV lasers are very powerful and can penetrate deep into tissue and often create a pleasant warming sensation over the area of treatment. Patients with chronic arthritis (i.e. knee pain) tend to respond well to these Class IV lasers.

Class IV lasers are generally used to work on many types of neuromuscular problems however they work especially well for treating neuropathies, chronic arthritis and stenosis conditions.

Class III are great for retraining muscles, stimulating nerves, breaking up adhesions, neuropathies and increasing overall function of the body.

Both of these lasers have value; however, each have their own particular strength. As a patient you should be able to expect at minimum:

- A decrease in pain (if not total elimination).
- A decrease in inflammation (swelling).

- A decrease need for pain medications.
- An increase in range of motion and muscle strength.
- As well as healing and repair of damaged tissues. This includes healing of bones, burns, sores, nerves, brain, tendons, ligaments and discs in the spine.

Laser is a phenomenal new treatment technology for healing old and new injuries. If there is an underlying mechanical cause for the pain, laser treatments are likely to give you safe and easy results.

What is Pulse Electro Magnetic Field Therapy (PEMF)

As far as celebrity doctors go, Dr. Oz has always been a favorite of mine because he's always looking for different ways to get you better without prescribing medications.

I may not agree with 100% of the things he says, but here is information from his show regarding pain and Pulse Electro-Magnetic Fields.

Pulsed Electro-Magnetic Fields or PEMF therapy has been used in Europe for over 30 years and has recently been brought over the US.

The National Institute of Health has made PEMFs a priority for research. In fact, many PEMF devices have already been approved by the FDA, some specifically to fuse broken bones, wound healing, pain and tissue swelling, and to treat depression. Most therapeutic PEMF devices are considered safe by various standards and organizations.

PEMFs work to:

- Decrease pain
- Reduce inflammation.
- Decrease the effects of stress on the body.
- Reduce platelet adhesion.
- Improved:
  - Energy
  - Circulation
  - Blood and tissue oxygenation
  - Sleep quality

- Blood pressure
- Cholesterol levels
- The uptake of nutrients
- Cellular detoxification
- Ability to regenerate cells
- Balances the immune system.
- Stimulates RNA and DNA.
- Accelerates repair of bone and soft tissue.
- Relaxes muscles.

What are PEMFs and how do they work?

Science teaches us that everything is energy. Energy is always dynamic and, therefore, has a frequency. It changes by the second or minute, for example, at the very least.

All energy is electromagnetic in nature. All atoms, chemicals and cells produce electromagnetic fields (EMFs).

Every organ in the body produces its own signature bioelectromagnetic field.

Science has proven that our bodies actually project their own magnetic fields and that all 70 trillion cells in the body communicate via electromagnetic frequencies. Nothing happens in the body without an electromagnetic exchange.

When the electromagnetic activity of the body ceases, life ceases. Just think about it, you need energy to absorb nutrients, heal up a wound, remove waste, communicate, etc.

As mentioned before we are electrical beings and each cell is a small, electrical battery that is conducting a current. When your battery is new and fully charged, good things tend to happen. However when your battery is older, like an old cell phone battery, the phone will not work as well and it will not last as long.

Pulsed electromagnetic field (PEMF) therapy is FDA-approved to fuse bones and has been cleared in certain devices to reduce swelling and joint pain.

This therapy has been used to treat pain and edema in soft tissue for over 60 years. The technology stemmed from radio frequency (RF) diathermy, which utilized a continuous electromagnetic field to produce heat in soft tissue.

A moving – or resonating – magnetic field can create currents without heating and thus directly alter cellular signaling.

It has been firmly established that tissues including blood, muscle, ligaments, bone and cartilage respond to biophysical input, including electrical and electromagnetic fields.

New studies show that with the proper field intensity and frequency, treatment with PEMF appears to be disease-modifying.

The stimulation of Transforming Growth Factor beta (TGF-beta) may be a mechanism by which PEMF favorably affects cartilage homeostasis. Through calcium-calmodulin-dependent pathways, PEMF may also increase nitric oxide activity.

Today many patients are seeking out this treatment for chronic pain. There are many devices out there today. Some are cheaper home units that cost a couple thousand. Higher end models are closer to $60,000 and are primarily used in medical offices.

The higher end models can deliver more power, penetrate deeper and provide quicker results.

Since the device uses electromagnetic frequencies, it is not indicated for patients with pacemakers, defibulators or cochlear implants or any device with a battery that cannot be removed.

Other than that side effects are minimal and the treatment results only take minutes to see.

Dr. Oz's episode can be found at www.desertpainrelief.com under the services tab called "PEMF."

Chapter 8: Secrets of the Far East

Acupuncture is one of the oldest healing arts in the world today. It originated in China and other Asian countries thousands of years ago.

Although it has gained much popularity in the US, some still perceive it as mysterious art. Acceptance in the US has grown since organizations like the Federal Drug Administration (FDA) and the National Institute of Health (NIH) have begun to perceive acupuncture as a type of medicine, rather than some sort of eccentric ritual.

As some Americans are losing patience with unsuccessful Western treatments, they are turning toward acupuncture.

Even celebrities are trying acupuncture and are reporting its benefits. Robert Downey Jr (Iron Man), Matt Damon, Gwyneth Paltrow, Kate Winslet, Kate Moss, Madonna, Neve Cambell and Cher are just some that have used acupuncture to help them with their health ailments. Many athletes are utilizing it for pain and a quicker recovery too!

Since it has no side effects or interactions with any other procedures, many team doctors welcome the ancillary procedure that will return their stars to the playing field as soon as possible.

Many of you already know someone who has received the benefits of acupuncture, but still do not know the theories behind it.

Acupuncture is a branch of Oriental Medicine that consists of the insertion of fine, sterile needles at specific acupoints on the body.

Traditional acupuncture is based on ancient Chinese theories of the flow of Qi (pronounced "chee").

Qi is the vital energy or life force in all living things that is necessary for growth, development, movement, maintenance of body temperature, and protection against illness and disease.

Qi flows along river-like meridians inside the body energizing, nourishing, and supporting every cell, tissue, muscle, organ and gland in the body.

In the Western view, acupuncture likely works by stimulating the central nervous system (the brain and spinal cord) to release chemicals called neurotransmitters, endorphins and hormones.

These chemicals dull pain, boost the immune system and regulate various body functions. Others believe that it is the regulation of blood flow that makes acupuncture work.

This has been well documented in some pain studies.

Some people say that it is difficult to perform a true randomized control study because of the placebo effect but studies have been done on animals.

Animals do not know if they are being treated for a particular injury, yet they still respond.

Today the majority of horse racers have acupuncture done on their horses for performance and pain management.

Traditional acupuncture involves placing needles at specific pressure points throughout the body.

Several different variations of this technique exist, however.

Some practitioners add heat or electrical stimulation to modify the treatment effects, while others substitute pressure for needles.

The needles are about the thickness of a hair so many people do not even feel the insertion.

Most people will feel the sensation like a mosquito bite during insertion and you may feel sensations such as warmth, a dull ache, tingling, heaviness, or a "moving" sensation. This is usually felt only for a short period of time, or if the practitioner is manipulating or stimulating the needle.

These are sensations of the needle connecting with your Qi.

Physical and emotional trauma, stress, lack of exercise, overexertion, seasonal changes, diet, accidents or excessive activity can lead to a blockage or imbalance of Qi.

When the disruption to Qi is prolonged or excessive, or if the body is in a weakened state, then illness, pain or disease may develop.

Many acupuncturists are also trained in Oriental Medicine, so they may prescribe Chinese herbs in addition to the acupuncture treatment.

According the World Health Organization (WHO), acupuncture works well with 47 known conditions, which is a broader band of therapy than anything else in the world.

Some of the popular conditions acupuncture treats are:

- Knee Pain
- Addiction
- Allergies
- Asthma
- Cosmetic Concerns
- Dental Pain
- Anxiety
- Depression
- Arthritis/Joint Pain
- Back And Neck Pain
- Carpal Tunnel Syndrome
- Effects Of Chemotherapy
- Erectile Dysfunction
- Fatigue
- Fibromyalgia
- Headaches
- Migraine
- Heartburn
- Indigestion
- Infertility
- Insomnia
- Menopause
- Menstrual Irregularities
- Nausea
- Numbness
- Neuropathy
- Sciatica
- Stroke Rehabilitation
- Tendonitis
- And Many More

Chapter 9: Hyaluronic Acid Joint Injections

Mistake #10: Skipping This Method Prior To Scheduling Surgery

Knee pain can be an excruciating and debilitating issue, especially when one experiences chronic discomfort in one or both knees as a result of complications related to osteoarthritis.

Poor quality of the natural substance known as hyaluronan located in the cartilage of the knee joint and the synovial fluid from which the joint receives support can result in the common symptoms of pain and immobility associated with osteoarthritis.

The role of this hyaluronan is one of cushioning and lubrication, so when it is not performing these roles at an optimum level of satisfaction, intervention may be required.

Intervening measures such as synvisc have traditionally been used to combat these issues, but a more effective, albeit more expensive solution exists.

Supartz is one of the purest forms of hyaluronic acid out of all the viscosupplement injections that leaves zero impurities when it is resorbed. Unlike synvisc which can cause inflammatory knee problems with repeat injections over time.

This therapeutic knee remedy involves the injection of a purified sodium hyaluronate solution known as hyaluronic acid which has been extracted from the combs of healthy roosters.

The result is the painful knee being supplemented with purified hyaluronan in order to counteract the issues related to osteoarthritis and helping to reduce the pain of the person suffering from this condition by acting to cushion and lubricate the knee joint.

The procedure is relatively quick and painless, starting with the prospective injection of a local anesthetic aimed to numb the knee from any potential discomfort experienced for the duration of the short procedure.

This procedure is really like changing the oil in your car or adding grease to a bearing.

It just provides a natural cushion to your joint, and Supartz is a thick protein that provides a natural cushion. The reason why it is not permanent is because your body will slowly eat away at the hyaluronic acid over time. This can last anywhere from 6 months to 2 years.

We have actually had patients who had it done 2 years ago and who have had no symptoms since. Factors that affect how long it lasts will be weight, use of knee and other biomechanical wear from factors mentioned earlier in the book.

The whole procedure can be done in the physician's office in a matter of minutes, and the recovery time is typically on the scale of hours, rather than weeks or months.

Our providers like to use a diagnostic ultrasound because it shows us what the joint looks like in real time. After 24 hours of avoiding strenuous activity following each injection, the patient should be able to go about their daily lives with greater mobility and less pain than they were previously experiencing before the supartz therapy took place.

This procedure is performed over 3 to 5 injections which will produce significant improvements in the quality of life and range of motion for most patients.

This procedure is extremely safe and studies have shown that it was no more dangerous than the placebo which was a salt water injection. The only problems noted were redness around the injection site from penetration of the skin with the needle.

Although this injection is relatively new in the US, it has been used in Europe for quite some time and there have been over 300 million injections worldwide.

Insurance companies like these types of procedures because they are relatively cheap and effective. In fact, Medicare and most major insurance companies cover this procedure. Even if you didn't have insurance, this procedure is still worthwhile for most for the effectiveness and cost factors involved.

Mistake #11: Not Utilizing Diagnostic Equipment

Some doctors prefer to inject blind, which means that they are feeling for the joint space by hand and injecting 'blind' meaning that they do not know what is under the skin.

It could be a vessel, nerve or a small joint space from arthritis build up. At our office we will typically have a digital radiograph (x-ray) as well as a diagnostic ultrasound that provides real time (live) viewing of the joint space.

Most doctors would prefer to use this equipment but since they are not medical devices, some Physicians choose to inject 'blind'.

Mistake #12: Unrealistic Expectations of Surgery

Although knee replacements have a very good success rate, it is always smart to try other therapies first before going under the knife.

Techniques in surgery are always improving and if you can maintain the quality of your life without chronic pain with these treatments, then I suggest you keep delaying your surgery.

Chapter 10: Platelet Rich Plasma

Platelet Rich Plasma Therapy (PRP) is a non-surgical treatment for soft tissue injuries and joint pain. PRP stimulates the body's natural healing forces.

Often a patient using PRP will be able to avoid more invasive procedures such as surgery. Chronic soft tissue injuries can be treated with PRP as an alternative to steroids.

What Is PRP?

PRP, or Platelet Rich Plasma, is a substance made from your own blood to trigger healing. Platelet Rich Plasma Therapy is a relatively simple, non-surgical treatment for joint injuries and arthritis. It merges cutting-edge technology with the body's natural ability to heal itself.

The PRP is a concentration of platelets, which can jump start healing. Platelets contain packets of growth hormones and cytokines that tell the tissues to increase rebuilding to enhance healing.

When PRP is injected into the damaged area, it stimulates a mild inflammatory response, which triggers the healing cascade.

This leads to restored blood flow, new cell growth, and tissue regeneration. This may ultimately result in faster healing of soft tissue injuries.

Where does PRP come from?

A sample of blood will be taken from a vein in your arm under sterile conditions. The blood will be placed in a centrifuge, which is a device that spins the blood.

This helps to separate the blood cells from the plasma, and allows concentration of the platelets. This concentration of platelets increases healing growth factors approximately 6 to 8 times greater than normal.

The preparation takes about 15 minutes. The finished PRP product is then available for injection into the injured joint or tendon under ultrasound guidance.

Because PRP is prepared from your own blood, there are no worries about rejection or disease transmission. In fact, PRP contains a high concentration of white blood cells, which helps to fight infection.

What are the potential benefits?

PRP enhances your healing potential. It is proving to often be an effective and natural alternative to steroid injections. Patients can see a significant improvement in symptoms as well as a remarkable return of function.

This may eliminate the need for more aggressive treatments such as long-term medication or surgery.

What Can I Expect During My Treatment?

You will visit with the doctor, who will ask about your medical history and give you a brief exam to determine that you are a good candidate for PRP therapy. We will obtain the blood sample and prepare the PRP.

The doctor will examine the area to be treated, sterilize the area, and apply numbing medicine.

Using ultrasound guidance, the PRP will be gently injected into the injured area and joint support tissues.

After your treatment, you will stay for a 15 to 20 minute observation period. At check-out, you will schedule a follow-up appointment and we will review discharge instructions.

The process may be repeated 1 to 2 times over a six to sixteen week period.

What Can I Expect After the PRP Treatment?

You may have mild to moderate discomfort which may last up to 1 week.

There may be temporary worsening of symptoms due to a stimulation of the inflammatory response, which is necessary for healing.

Your doctor will instruct you in the use of ice, elevation, reduced activity, and analgesic medications for comfort while the PRP is initiating healing.

Also physical therapy or a therapeutic exercise program will be prescribed.

What Should I Do When I Get Home Following the Procedure?

Because Platelet Rich Plasma releases growth factors, it is important to not disturb the area of injection for at least 48 hours.

We ask that you refrain from activities other than necessary walking or driving in order to receive the maximum benefit of the PRP growth factor stimulation.

It is helpful if you can be sedentary for 48 hours, and refrain from any vigorous activity for up to 2 weeks following each procedure.

Mistake #13: No Personal Attention

This one is not so much a mistake, but more of a trend with specialists. In the new age of electronic medical records, as a provider it requires us to focus on a tablet or computer screen while taking our notes.

We all have families and finishing up medical notes on a patient at lunch or after work sucks, but I started in my field because I had a great experience with my doctor that saved me from surgery.

I am a little old fashioned but I think that the relationship and energy with the patient is part of the healing as well.

I believe in looking people in the eye, putting my hands on the patient and really listening to their concerns. With these new medical note taking systems it requires us to focus on the computer rather than the patient and I often hear patients complain about the specialist who sat in the corner with their back to them while typing at their computer.

I personally detest this but found myself doing it when I upgraded to my medical note taking system.

I hated it, however, and so I hired a medical assistant to be in charge of charting notes for our medical staff so they can focus on taking care of you and not the computer screen.

This is a small added cost to our office, but I believe that the extra personal attention will make you feel better about your procedure.

People in pain can be irritable and definitely anxious when new procedures are performed on their knee. Personal attention makes the experience easier.

After all, this is why we got into healthcare, to take care of people and not to ignore them when they are in need. We like to think of ourselves as servants in the office and patients like you are the ones we serve.

Mistake #14: Treating Services Like Commodities.

All too often I will have patients price shop treatments thinking that all types of the same treatment should be the same across the board.

This is true if you are buying a commodity such medication, wheel chairs or bandages but it is not the same with human services.

As far as comparing treatments from provider to provider like a commodity...good luck. In general, you typically get what you pay for and you can't go to the cheapest surgeon in town and expect the best results.

This is not always the case, but you definitely cannot price shop for a type of service.

You have to find the person who is caring, trusting, gets the job done and hopefully at a fair price. Fair doesn't mean cheap, it just means for the results, expertise and service that it is a fair price.

Chapter 11: Custom Made Braces Outperform A One Size Fits All Brace

When excessive pain or discomfort, or even simply a lack of mobility of the knee joint necessitates a knee brace, making the right choice is crucial.

Many cheap and generic knee braces exist which can be purchased relatively inexpensively from drug stores everywhere.

These are typically made of neoprene or some other type of cheap material which generally provides little support beyond a bit of compression to compact the tissues in and around the knee.

While potentially helpful in some situations, braces such as these are generally not ideal.

Serving more as a temporary bandage of sorts, they fail to solve any of the issues which necessitated the brace in the first place.

Whether these issues are due to a single traumatic event that caused a severe injury, repetitive stress, or chronic issues like varying types of arthritis, custom braces are generally much more effective than their generic neoprene counterparts.

Custom models offer much greater support due to their hinged design. They fit better because they are specifically crafted to fit your leg and support your knee. They are bigger and bulkier but in this case these factors are a good thing because they afford the support that your knee needs.

If one or both of your knees are bad enough to require a brace, you are better off choosing the brace that's going to be the most effective for you. Custom hinged models can be more comfortable to wear for prolonged periods of time relative to the neoprene models which may prove to be too tight when worn for too long.

Most importantly, the hinged models that can be made custom to fit each individual simply work better in that they provide the proper support where it is needed most.

There are only four main ligaments in the knee that must support and control the knee joint. The Knee joint itself needs to support all of the body mass above it which is constantly being pulled down by gravity onto the knees.

Any brace used on the knee needs to work well to provide the required support.

It is the custom hinged models of knee braces which focus the support on the right areas, taking stress off of the medial and lateral portions of the knee. On the inner side of the knee (proximal to the midline of the body) is the medial collateral ligament (MCL).

On the opposite side (distal to the midline of the body), the lateral collateral ligament provides support on the outer side of the knee.

The custom models of knee braces which feature a hinged design are able to provide support to both of this areas, ensuring that both the inner and outer sides of the knee joint are supported by the brace.

It is generally the medial or lateral portions of the knee which feature the greatest arthritic concern for patients suffering from some type of arthritis, so this added support in these areas is a welcome addition afforded by the custom hinged models.

The generic neoprene models are unable to offer this level of performance.

If you are looking for a knee brace then make sure you consider opting for a custom model with a hinged design over a simple neoprene one which may be cheaper but also less effective.

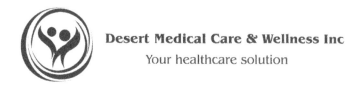

Desert Medical Care & Wellness Inc
Your healthcare solution

Chapter 12 :Mistake #15 - Not Using This Checklist to Help You Find a Doctor or Therapist That Will Take Care Of You

Checklist:

- ☐ Is there any diagnostic equipment used for your diagnosis such as x-ray, MRI, CT scan, ultrasound, etc. If not, why was it not used?
- ☐ Does this office offer solutions like foam rolling and a therapy stick for adhesions in the muscles causing pain?
- ☐ Does this office offer pre-digested joint supplements? Does this office understand that glucosamine, MSM, chondroitin and herbs are difficult for

people over the age of 50 to break down and make bioavailable?

☐ Did the doctor assess if my pelvis, hips, glutes, ankles and other areas were involved in my knee pain? Do they offer orthotics or knee braces if I need them?

☐ Does my pain come from the same type of activity over and over again? If so, what methods are used to address this?

☐ Does the Chiropractor offer other high tech options for joint manipulation other than 'manually popping' the joints if I am anxious about it? If not, why not?

☐ Does my Chiropractor only offer 'joint manipulation' for my condition or is there exercise and muscle therapy?

☐ Does this clinic offer deep tissue Class IV laser and PEMF therapy for knee pain and arthritis?

☐ Does this clinic offer the option of acupuncture, chiropractic, massage and physiotherapy?

☐ Does this office offer dietary counseling and weight loss methods that can achieve 12-25 pounds per month? Do they offer weekly dietary counseling and weigh-ins at a minimal onetime fee? Do they offer metabolism booster injections?

☐ Am I getting substandard care because of my insurance?

☐ Does this office offer alternative injections to cortisone such as hyaluronic acid injections?

☐ Does this office use digital x-rays and diagnostic ultrasound for joint injections?

☐ Is surgery considered to be the cure-all for my condition? Is it worth the risk and have I tried all conservative therapies before I tried this last and final one?

☐ Am I just taking pain pills/shots for my condition and just covering up the symptoms temporarily?

☐ Does my Doctor even care about me? Do they look me in the eye when they speak or do they just sit in the corner typing on their computer?

- ☐ Do I believe that all Doctors are equal at what they do?
- ☐ Do they offer a 5 point system for knee pain relief?
- ☐ Proper diagnostic imaging with orthopedic examination and ultrasound guided knee injections.
- ☐ Complete structure assessment, treatment and rehabilitation program that includes: foot/ankle, knee, hip/pelvis and non-effected side. This includes soft tissue and joint mobilization and lower body rehabilitation.
- ☐ Deep tissue laser therapy, PEMF and acupuncture for pain and healing
- ☐ Hyaluronic acid knee injection
- ☐ Pre-digested, 100% bio-available joint supplements (only one in the USA, so you probably are not taking it unless you purchased it from our office).

Conclusion

We've talked about many different keys to non-surgical knee pain treatment. Make sure to take action on what you've discovered in these chapters.

Just to recap, you learned why alignment matters and how a pelvic, hip, ankle or foot alignment problem could lead to excessive wear on the knee joint and eventually arthritis.

You learned why balancing the pelvic muscles and breaking up adhesions in the muscle can alleviate or cure your knee pain.

You learned about hyaluronic acid injections, PRP, custom made braces, physiotherapy, chiropractic, laser, PEMF and acupuncture for pain control.

You learned how a simple 10% reduction in body weight can alleviate your knee pain as well.

You learned why taking Ibprofen, Aleve, Tylenol along with cortisone shots only makes things worse in the long run.

You learned why surgery, even though successful in most cases, should be avoided until you have tried alternatives listed in this book.

To conclude, I'll leave you with the #1 secret for achieving long term change: *You simply take one healthy step at a time.*

I know you were looking for the silver bullet, but correcting these problems allows you to have success when you thought surgery was inevitable.

Basically, it boils down to becoming

accountable for your health because your health is your number one asset.

You have control of this every day when you wake up, from dawn until dusk.

It's only about pursuing long lasting change, and taking accountability for your health so you can free yourself from your knee pain and get long lasting results

I hope this information helps you, but the best solution is to get a recommendation from an expert in non-surgical knee treatment.

This treatment can't help everyone and sometimes we are just prolonging surgery.

This is why we offer a free consultation because we don't want there to be any cost issues holding you back from learning how you could avoid surgery with this new and unique treatment combination.

During our office visit, you will have a 1-on-1 appointment with me please fill out your patient paperwork found on www.DesertKneePain.com that will provide us the information we need to make a recommendation.

This visit should take no more than 30 minutes, but this 30 minutes could be the answer to your knee pain problem that you have been waiting for.

No more elevators because stairs will be no problem when you are done with our program.

If you would like to call us directly for an appointment please call 760-209-5655 to set up your free life changing appointment today.

In Health,

Dr. Olesnicky, MD & Dr. Hashimoto, DC

Index

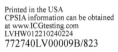

9 781508 441434